Health consequences of the Chernobyl accident

Results of the IPHECA pilot projects and related national programmes

Summary Report

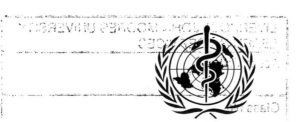

World Health Organization
Geneva

WHO Library Cataloguing in Publication Data

Health consequences of the Chernobyl accident : results of the IPHECA pilot projects
        and related national programmes : summary report.

    1.Nuclear medicine.   2.Accidents, Radiation   3.Radiation effects   4.Radiation monitoring

    ISBN 92 4 156181 5   (NLM Classification: WN 440)

© World Health Organization 1995

PRINTED IN SWITZERLAND
95/10668 – Atar – 10 000

Contents

Foreword

In 1986 an explosion occurred at the Chernobyl nuclear power plant in the former Soviet Union. Shock and fear quickly spread around the world together with the news of the threat of radiation. The Chernobyl explosion had released a radioactive cloud which passed over a number of countries, leading governments to take a variety of measures to protect the health of their populations.

Immediately after the accident, in collaboration with the government of the former Soviet Union, many initiatives were taken by the relevant organizations, including WHO and other international agencies. In 1991, WHO's participation in this effort was formalized through the official establishment of the International Programme on the Health Effects of the Chernobyl Accident (IPHECA). This Programme is a cooperative initiative of WHO, the governments of Belarus, the Russian Federation and Ukraine, and a number of other countries and institutions.

The areas most contaminated by radiation from the Chernobyl accident are in Belarus, the Russian Federation and Ukraine, where Chernobyl is located. In addition to the effects of radiation, many people in the contaminated areas also suffered the stress of extreme fear and the disruption of forced evacuation which have affected both their physical and their mental health. Massive efforts have been made by these three countries to reduce potential health damage, to provide diagnosis, treatment and rehabilitation to those affected and to investigate the effects on health which have occurred. Considerable resources have been expended in supporting these efforts. In this regard, a major role of IPHECA over the past few years has been to strengthen the capacity of national health care institutions by providing medical equipment and by training staff in diagnosis and treatment and in modern techniques of data collection and analysis.

Almost ten years have passed since the Chernobyl accident, but the work of monitoring the health effects and assisting those affected is still going on. The accident exposed large numbers of people to low levels of radiation over an extended period of time. Continuing study of the health of these populations will improve scientific understanding of the effects of radiation and indicate how best to help those whose health has been impaired. Maximum benefit can be achieved only through international cooperation, as continued investigation and progress in health care also require continued financial support and demonstration of solidarity betweeen all countries and peoples.

This report summarizes a much more extensive one, entitled *Health consequences of the Chernobyl accident. Results of the IPHECA pilot projects and related national programmes: scientific report.*[1] The major contributors to the full report are the specialist staff of the institutes concerned with the aftermath of the accident in Belarus, the Russian Federation and Ukraine. They include the project managers, doctors and scientists who have worked relentlessly on investigating and mitigating the health consequences of the accident every day and, for many of them, since the first days after the explosion. Their first-hand experience, their knowledge and their dedicated work are extremely valuable.

I believe sincerely that IPHECA's efforts to assist national governments have helped in alleviating the anguish and the suffering caused by the Chernobyl accident. This report describes what has been done and gives a glimpse of the enormous work of monitoring health and collecting and analysing data that must continue for years to come. The Programme has already generated a vast amount of knowledge about the health effects of a nuclear accident on the general population, and more knowledge will be forthcoming in future. It is our responsibility to ensure that this knowledge can be used for the benefit of all. If ever a massive release of radiation were to occur again, we must be ready to respond in a way that would save the lives and protect the health of as many people as possible.

As an essential contribution to nuclear emergency preparedness, IPHECA must remain an integral part of a comprehensive policy for the prevention of nuclear accidents. Preparedness and prevention cannot be dissociated from each other. Let us never forget that nuclear risk is shared by all, and that prevention and preparedness against such risk must therefore be jointly ensured by all.

Hiroshi Nakajima, M.D., Ph.D.
Director-General
World Health Organization

---

[1] See footnote on facing page.

Introduction

The largest-ever radiation accident involving a nuclear reactor occurred on 26 April 1986 at the Chernobyl nuclear power plant in Ukraine. Heavy contamination spread over large areas of Belarus, the Russian Federation and Ukraine. The Chernobyl accident killed 30 of the workers at the reactor site, caused the hospitalization of hundreds of others and exposed five million people to ionizing radiation caused by fallout of radioactive nuclides. This has led so far to a large increase in thyroid cancer among children in affected areas. Other signs of health deterioration in these areas require further investigation.

WHO's International Programme on the Health Effects of the Chernobyl Accident (IPHECA) was established to support national programmes, monitor health consequences and indicate future work needed to ensure that maximum information is gained from this disaster. IPHECA has been in operation since 1991 and has been supported by contributions from the Czech Republic, Finland, Japan, Slovakia and Switzerland. There have been substantial inputs from the governments of Belarus, the Russian Federation and Ukraine which provided clinical facilities, personnel and financial support and created the conditions necessary for the successful implementation of the Programme. This report describes IPHECA's work and gives details on the extent of radionuclide contamination and the responses by the three national authorities and various international agencies. It summarizes the longer report, *Health consequences of the Chernobyl accident. Results of the IPHECA pilot projects and related national programmes: scientific report.*[1]

Levels of radioactive contamination are given in this report in kilobecquerels per square metre (kBq/m^2). The becquerel (Bq) is the unit by which radioactivity is measured and is equal to one atomic disintegration per second (1 kBq = 1000 atomic disintegrations per second).

Exposure is measured in millisieverts. The millisievert (mSv) is a unit of radiation dose equivalent to about 50 general chest X-rays. On average, people are naturally exposed to about 1 mSv a year from background radiation, which comes from traces of radioactive isotopes that occur in all natural and man-made materials. However, there are many locations around the world where

---

[1] Unpublished WHO document WHO/EHG/95.19, in preparation. For further information, contact the Office of Global and Integrated Environmental Health, World Health Organization, CH-1211 Geneva 27, Switzerland.

1

people are naturally exposed to higher concentrations of radioactive materials, causing exposures up to 10 mSv a year. Table 1 shows natural background ionizing radiation levels (to which everything is exposed), levels at which health effects may occur and the levels for which radiation protection standards have been established.

Table 1

Radiation doses and possible consequences from whole-body exposure

Typical annual dose of natural background	Dose in areas of high natural background	Lowest single dose for health effects	Approximate single dose for radiation sickness	Single dose, survival unlikely
1 mSv	10 mSv	200 mSv	1000 mSv	10 000 mSv

International Commission on Radiological Protection effective dose limit per year for exposures above natural background: public, 1 mSv; workers, 5 mSv.

1

The accident

The Chernobyl power station had four nuclear reactors, each housed in a separate unit. On the night of 25–26 April 1986 the staff of Unit 4 were testing a turbogenerator just prior to shutting the reactor down. According to the report of the International Chernobyl Project, coordinated by the International Atomic Energy Agency (IAEA), test procedures were poorly written and operating rules were disregarded with the result that staff disabled many of the safety systems and withdrew control rods from the reactor's core. Because of this, a huge power surge that occurred in the reactor did not trigger an automatic shutdown, as it normally should have done, and could not be controlled manually.

At 01:23 on 26 April the reactor in Unit 4 exploded, cutting its cooling channels. A few seconds later a second explosion destroyed part of the building and threw hot and highly radioactive pieces of the reactor core into the air. Burning graphite fell on several nearby buildings and started fires.

Destruction of the reactor's housing released large amounts of radioactive materials into the atmosphere. After the explosions, entry of air and radioactive fission kept the graphite core burning. In the days that followed, some 5000 tonnes of boron, dolomite, sand, clay and lead were dropped on Unit 4 to put out the fire and reduce the fission reaction. These materials initially insulated the reactor core and even made the temperature increase. Further, the process of dropping the materials on the reactor caused plumes of particles to be thrown into the air, adding to the radioactive cloud that was forming. By 5 May the reactor began to cool down and the release of radioactivity started to subside.

Radioactive contamination

It has been estimated that the total radioactivity of the material released from the reactor was 200 times that of the combined releases from the atomic bombs dropped on Hiroshima and Nagasaki.

There was initially high radiation exposure for the firemen from the towns of Pripyat and Chernobyl who were called to put out the fires started by the radioactive debris. The staff of the power plant itself were of course also exposed to high levels of radioactivity as they carried out emergency operations.

Subsequently, accident recovery workers, both civilian and military, were drafted in by the authorities to decontaminate the power plant and surrounding area. They also helped build the enormous sarcophagus in which the reactor was eventually buried to prevent further contamination. These workers were deployed for only short periods and were regularly replaced because of the high radiation exposure. It is estimated that 800 000 people were involved in this work altogether.

The radionuclides in the cloud over Chernobyl were mainly iodine-131, caesium-134 and caesium-137. The cloud was dispersed by the wind and the nuclides were deposited as fallout over large areas of the Soviet Union and other parts of the northern hemisphere. The first indication of the accident outside the USSR was the detection of increased levels of radioactivity in Finland and Sweden two days later.

High concentrations of radioactive materials were deposited by rainfall in areas close to the reactor. The radioisotope with the greatest effect on health initially was iodine-131 which accumulates in the thyroid. This isotope has a half-life of eight days, so its effect is short-term. The radioactive nuclide causing most long-term exposure was caesium-137, which has a half-life of 30 years. Caesium contamination in excess of 555 kBq/m² covered some 10 000 km², while a further 21 000 km² had contamination of 185–555 kBq/m². In Belarus, about 20% of the population (2.2 million people) live in areas where there was contamination of more than 37 kBq/m².

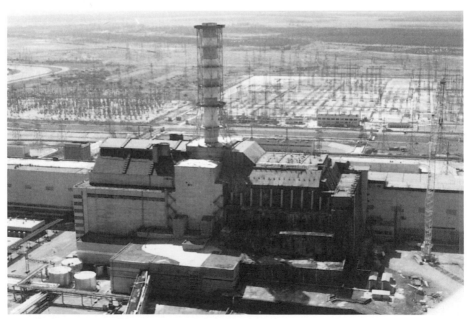

The Chernobyl nuclear reactor number 4 enclosed in its sarcophagus (photo IAEA/ V. Mouchkin).

2

Response by national authorities

When details of the accident became known, a government commission was set up to coordinate the activities of the departments and ministries of the three Soviet republics and the work of the medical institutions giving assistance to the affected population. A medical commission was set up soon afterwards.

Following the Chernobyl accident, the Soviet authorities classified zones of radioactive contamination as follows:

- 37–555 kBq/m²   periodic health monitoring, no special measures adopted;
- 555–1480 kBq/m²   strict control, restrictions imposed on population, restrictions on use of locally produced food, decontamination measures adopted;
- over 1480 kBq/m²   area classified as unfit for human habitation, population evacuated.

On the basis of this classification, the medical commission set a 30-km limit for evacuation around Chernobyl. Some 135 000 people living within 30 km of the reactor were consequently evacuated to less heavily contaminated areas. The town of Pripyat (pop. 45 000) was the largest population centre to be evacuated. This was done on 27 April, 36 hours after the accident, and took only three hours once the decision to evacuate had been taken. At the time of the Chernobyl accident more than 400 000 people lived in the areas contaminated with more than 555 kBq/m², which are known as Strictly Controlled Zones. Some 270 000 people still live in these areas. Table 2 shows the different actions taken by the Soviet authorities according to levels of contamination caused by the accident.

Registration and medical follow-up are compulsory for four main groups of persons: accident recovery workers, persons evacuated from areas contaminated with more than 1480 kBq/m², persons resident in areas contaminated with 555–1480 kBq/m², and the children of persons in these groups.

One of the initial concerns of the medical commission was to reduce the potential health hazard of radioiodine to the population, and above all to children. The situation was complicated by the variations in the radioiodine fallout pattern. Potassium iodide or iodate tablets were provided for 5.3 million people, of whom 1.6 million were children. The first to receive this treatment were those evacuated from the 30-km zone.

The Soviet Ministry of Health approved a provisional accident regulation that set maximum permissible radioisotope concentrations in milk (3700 Bq per litre), dairy products, fish, meat, bread, vegetables and other foods. An

5

Table 2

Population exposed to radioactive contamination and actions taken by the Soviet authorities

Levels of contamination per m²	Average exposure rate per year	Population exposed	Action taken
over 1480 kBq	over 5 mSv	135 000	All evacuated
555–1480 kBq	up to 5 mSv	270 000	Helped to relocate if requested, compulsory health monitoring
185–555 kBq	up to 2 mSv	580 000	Special health monitoring
37–185 kBq	up to 1 mSv	4 000 000	Regular health monitoring

immediate ban was placed on the consumption of milk and other foodstuffs contaminated above the maximum permissible level. These restrictions were generally effective, but in some localities (and especially among some of the rural population) the restrictions were not observed, or only partly implemented.

A number of the former Soviet Union's specialized institutes began large-scale investigations of the thyroid and this research has since been continued under national programmes. However, acute shortages of modern medical equipment, particularly for ultrasonic verification of the size and structure of the thyroid, inevitably meant that some medical information could not be obtained.

Since the half-life of iodine-131 is only eight days, the danger from radioiodine declined considerably within a few months. As that threat reduced, increased attention was paid to whole-body radiation doses. The Ministry of Health introduced a regulation, approved by the government commission, which set 100 mSv as the maximum permissible accidental whole-body radiation dose during the first year after the accident. The maximum limit was reduced to 30 mSv for the second year and was later lowered to 25 mSv per year for 1988 and 1989. Consequently, over the four years following the accident, the total dose burden per person was not to exceed 180 mSv. However, it was virtually impossible for the regulation to be fully complied with among such large population groups and therefore some individuals received larger doses. The USSR's National Commission for Radiation Protection (NCRP) recommended 350 mSv as the lifetime dose limit for external and internal irradiation from the Chernobyl accident. Compliance with the limit was monitored in a representative group for each settlement, but monitoring of the highest individual doses also became increasingly important. The established limits became the basis for continuing or discontinuing protective measures in individual settlements, and especially for deciding whether or not to evacuate inhabitants from areas where it would have been impossible to enforce the regulations.

6

In 1990 the Supreme Soviet of Belarus declared the entire republic an ecological disaster zone. Medical personnel were hired to assist health care institutions in the affected localities. A medical college was opened in Gomel and students who agreed to work in the contaminated areas after graduation were recruited.

In the Medical Radiological Research Centre at Obninsk, the Russian State Medical and Radiological Registry was established soon after the accident for persons affected by radiation. A diagnostic centre was set up and equipped in Bryansk, the most affected oblast.[1] Also in that oblast, a branch of the St Petersburg Institute of Radiation Hygiene was established in the town of Novozybkov. Local medical care institutions were supplied by the government with modern diagnostic facilities and extra medical staff. In hospitals in the rayons,[2] new departments were created for medical monitoring, social and psychological rehabilitation and dosimetry control. Twenty-eight whole-body counters and facilities for thermoluminescent dosimetry were set up in dosimetry services in Bryansk and Kaluga oblasts, and guidelines were provided for dose reconstruction (retrospective estimation of dose received). Medical teams from leading scientific institutions and local hospitals worked in the affected areas and scientific data were collected for thorough analysis.

In Ukraine, the Ministry of Health allocated additional resources to medical assistance in the days immediately after the accident. Despite the extremely complex radiation pattern, a preliminary forecast of the population's annual external and internal radiation doses was developed as early as June 1986. Protective measures for limiting intake of radionuclides through food and water were introduced in an effort to reduce the forecast irradiation levels. Outpatient clinics were set up in the city of Kiev for the identification, registration and observation of persons exposed to radiation and for provision of treatment and consultation services. An All-Union Research Centre of Radiation Medicine and a Scientific Council for Radiation Medicine were established to conduct scientific analyses and to coordinate follow-up action concerning different population groups. Technical and software support were supplied to the All-Union and Republic Distributed Medical and Dosimetry Registry and to specialized subregistries to facilitate long-term observations.

The health authorities are continuing to monitor the health of the affected population and record the results in the appropriate registries. The annex on page 37 gives a chronology of the Chernobyl accident, listing the main developments that followed.

---

[1] Oblast – a large territorial and administrative division. Each country consists of a number of oblasts.

[2] Rayon – a smaller territorial and administrative division. Each oblast consists of a number of rayons.

3

Activities of international organizations

Many international bodies, both within and outside the United Nations, have been involved in the evaluation and alleviation of the medical effects of the Chernobyl accident. WHO's Regional Office for Europe played a major role immediately after the accident. Despite the complexity of the situation and lack of available information, the Regional Office was able to make sound, well accepted recommendations on what actions were necessary to protect health in the region. While monitoring of foodstuffs, especially milk, was recommended to Member States outside the Soviet Union, it was considered unnecessary to keep people indoors, ban the use of groundwater for drinking, or use iodine prophylaxis. Subsequently WHO and the Food and Agriculture Organization of the United Nations (FAO) were involved in defining maximum levels of radioactivity in food for consumption.

IAEA was asked by the Soviet Government to coordinate an international assessment of the radiological consequences of the accident and the criteria used for protecting the population. This was known as the International Chernobyl Project. IAEA led an inter-agency assessment (in which WHO participated) of the early radiological consequences of the accident during 1990 and 1991. This gave a comprehensive picture of the environmental and health situation in the affected areas at the time. The outcome of the project was important for the development of future work in this field.

The United Nations Scientific Committee on the Effects of Atomic Radiation (UNSCEAR) published a comprehensive assessment of worldwide contamination from the accident in 1988. A subsequent report is being drafted.

The United Nations Educational, Scientific and Cultural Organization (UNESCO) has been involved in several areas of assistance, namely the social and psychological rehabilitation of children, the social and economic aspects of resettlement of populations, the production of prefabricated housing, and the training of interpreters.

The Commission of the European Communities has facilitated scientific meetings and research in the contaminated areas, as well as treatment of accident victims, training of medical staff and provision of medical equipment. Research has included biological dosimetry for dose reconstruction and epidemiological investigations, particularly on thyroid cancer. This has been carried out in collaboration with the International Agency for Research on Cancer and the WHO Regional Office for Europe.

A number of other international organizations, national institutions and foundations from various countries have done, and continue to do, valuable work in many communities of the three countries. They include the International Federation of Red Cross and Red Crescent Societies, the Sasakawa Foundation, the Franco-Ukrainian Centre and many others.

4

The International Programme on the Health Effects of the Chernobyl Accident (IPHECA)

Between 1986 and 1989, WHO collaborated with the authorities in the USSR on a series of activities related to the Chernobyl accident. In early 1990 this collaboration led to a proposal by the Ministry of Health of the USSR that WHO develop an international programme to mitigate the health consequences of the accident. Over the next year a number of expert consultations were convened by WHO to elaborate the programme and to identify priorities.

The WHO Executive Board and the World Health Assembly reviewed the development of the programme in 1991. In May 1991 the World Health Assembly, in Resolution WHA44.36, officially endorsed the establishment of IPHECA under the auspices of WHO. Practical details were laid down in an agreement signed by the ministers of health of Belarus, the Russian Federation and Ukraine, and the Director-General of WHO in April 1992.

IPHECA is a cooperative effort of the three affected countries, WHO, including the Regional Office for Europe, and a number of other countries and organizations (Fig. 1). Its broad aim is to support efforts to relieve the health consequences of the accident by assisting health authorities in the affected countries, and especially in areas significantly contaminated by radionuclides

Fig. 1

Organizational structure of IPHECA

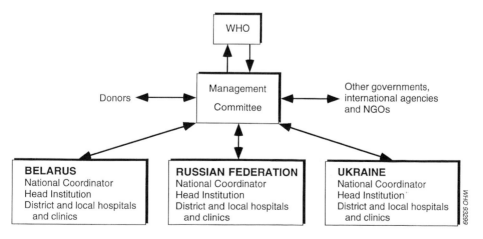

11

(Fig. 2), through provision of equipment, training and expert advice and exchange of information. IPHECA's other objectives are to consolidate experience gained from treatment of radiation exposure and from various practical interventions, thereby improving medical preparedness for the future, and to acquire data on the epidemiology of radiation-related health effects.

Management and resources

Responsibility for the overall management of IPHECA was vested in its management committee. This comprised representatives of Belarus, the Russian Federation, Ukraine, WHO and Member States of the Organization who had donated funds to the programme. Other cooperating parties attended meetings of the management committee as observers.

The functions of the committee included:
- reviewing and approving annual workplans;
- ensuring that the programme's work was subject to independent scientific review;
- promoting coordination of all relevant Chernobyl health-related projects.

The committee has met annually under the chairmanship of WHO. It was assisted by ad hoc scientific advisory bodies which reviewed IPHECA's progress, discussed scientific problems and ensured the scientific validity of all decisions.

Fig. 2

Region covered by IPHECA

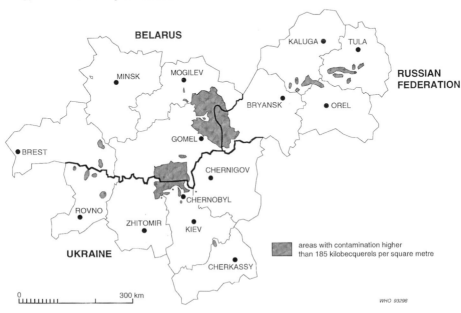

IPHECA has been implemented through the combined efforts of institutions at different levels (national, oblast, rayon). Some 200 professional staff in the three countries contributed to this work. Each country designated a national IPHECA coordinator with responsibility for ensuring that the work was carried out efficiently and effectively. In addition, a leading institution in each country took responsibility for all aspects of the programme within the country. The national coordinators and supervisory institutions were as follows:

- Belarus
  Minister of Health
  Research Institute for Radiation Medicine, Minsk
- Russian Federation
  Director
  Medical Radiological Research Centre, Obninsk
- Ukraine
  Vice-Minister of Health
  Ukrainian Research Centre for Radiation Medicine, Kiev.

In WHO, a senior radiation scientist was responsible for day-to-day implementation of IPHECA. Other scientific and administrative staff gave support in the areas of training and the procurement of equipment and supplies.

The resources received for IPHECA amount to over US$20 000 000. In addition to the major contribution from Japan, financial support was provided by the Czech Republic, Finland, Slovakia and Switzerland. Support also came from institutions in France, Germany, Japan and the United Kingdom who trained personnel or took part in scientific exchanges. Substantial national budgets were devoted to IPHECA activities by the three affected countries.

5

Types of health consequences

The health consequences of the Chernobyl accident are complex. While preliminary results are available it will take many years before the full extent of the accident's effects on health is known and complete data on the health consequences are in a form that can be properly analysed and validated. IPHECA has helped build the infrastructure that will facilitate study of the health effects. While some effects on health are due to direct radiation exposure, others may be a consequence of non-radiation factors.

Non-radiation effects

People in the affected areas naturally feared that they had been exposed to radiation that might cause future health damage. This fear was made worse by the lack of information immediately after the accident. WHO addressed this issue by publishing and distributing 100 000 booklets on the accident for people in the affected areas. Written in Russian for non-specialists, the booklets gave straightforward information about the effects of radiation on health. One of the principal objectives was to allay fears about the effects of radiation exposure. It was stated, for instance, that the vast majority of people would suffer no radiation-induced effects because the doses they received were very low. While it was not possible to measure the success of the booklet in allaying people's fears, it was recognized that the psychological impact of the accident was a major health effect that needed to be addressed.

Another psychological problem related to the evacuation of people from the most contaminated regions. When people are evacuated from their homes, they often suffer considerable stress because they do not have full information about what is going on, they undergo disruption in community infrastructure and social interaction, and they face uncertainty about housing and employment. Many evacuees who moved to new settlements after the Chernobyl accident were particularly depressed in their new homes because of financial difficulties, fear of isolation, and concern for the health of their children. Many people living in areas of less contamination were not evacuated but their daily activities were subject to a wide range of restrictions, especially with regard to food and water, designed to keep down the level of radiation exposure. The tense situation caused considerable stress which, combined with the constant fear of health damage from the radioactive fallout, led to a rising number of health disorders being reported to local outpatient clinics.

15

The immediate psychological impact of the accident on people in the affected areas was similar to that of a natural disaster such as earthquake, fire or flood. A psychological and clinical survey conducted after the accident showed that headaches, a feeling of pressure in the chest, indigestion, sleep disturbance, irritability, loss of concentration and abuse of alcohol were common. Although the countermeasures following the accident reduced radiation doses, they increased tension and the upheavals resulted in significant psychological stress in the affected population.

Aside from the reports of symptoms or signs of ill-defined conditions, the health registries recorded large increases in a number of specific diseases, especially in children. These have included endocrine diseases, mental disorders, and diseases of the nervous system, sensory organs, and digestive and genitourinary systems. Congenital abnormalities have also been observed. While present evidence does not suggest that these diseases are radiation-induced, it is possible that additional diseases and medical problems may have resulted from the considerable stress that people experienced.

Radiation effects

Radiation has both immediate health effects such as radiation sickness and longer-term effects such as thyroid cancer and leukaemia. The probability of suffering these longer-term effects increases with the amount of radiation exposure. The immediate effects of the accident were limited to reactor plant personnel and firemen called in to extinguish the graphite fire. Two died during the accident, one from severe burns and one was never found in the debris. When the accident occurred, 444 people were at the reactor site and were exposed to large amounts of radiation. Some 300 were admitted to hospitals and 134 were diagnosed as having acute radiation sickness (108 in Moscow, 26 in Kiev). Twenty-eight of these died within the first three months. Of the workers who recovered from acute radiation sickness, most continued with emotional and sleep disturbances. Some 30% of these workers suffered various disorders (gastrointestinal, cardiovascular, immune function) that reduced their ability to work. No clinical symptoms of acute radiation syndrome were seen in the people evacuated from the 30-km zone or in residents of the affected areas.

Radioactive iodine (predominantly iodine-131), with a half-life of eight days, was the most important radionuclide during the first few weeks after the accident. When iodine is absorbed by the body either through inhalation or in food, it accumulates mainly in the thyroid. Many people in the affected areas around Chernobyl had a shortage of iodine in their diet so their bodies would absorb iodine readily. More than five million people are reported to have received non-radioactive iodine tablets (to block absorption of radioactive iodine from the fallout) as a protective measure, but large numbers of children did not receive these tablets. Thus some people, especially children, received large radiation doses to the thyroid, resulting in an increase in thyroid disorders, particularly cancer.

Radioactive caesium irradiates the body either through contaminated food or by direct external exposure to contaminated materials such as soil, buildings and clothing. In the first year after the accident, much of the caesium radioactivity was found on the green parts of plants. Later, as radiocaesium was absorbed into the soil, radioactivity entered the food chain via vegetables and via plants eaten by animals. Drinking-water was contaminated, resulting in further radiation exposure.

Because of the different ways in which people can be exposed to radiation and the different parts of the body affected by each radionuclide, the range of potential health problems is wide. Aside from the acute radiation effects of large exposures and the potential for thyroid diseases from radioiodine, follow-up of the survivors of the atomic bombs dropped on Hiroshima and Nagasaki suggested that late radiation effects such as leukaemia and other blood diseases also needed to be studied. In addition, there was the likelihood of damage to the fetus, especially if mothers were exposed to radiation at the critical stage of pregnancy when the fetal organs are beginning to form. Brain damage *in utero* is of special interest and can be measured as a deficit in intellect or detected as behavioural and emotional disorders.

6

Results of the IPHECA pilot projects on health consequences

The Chernobyl accident resulted in a wide range of both actual and potential health problems. Solutions to these problems were seen to require the following:
- diagnosis, treatment and, where possible, prevention of the health effects of the accident and its aftermath;
- alleviation of the adverse social and psychological consequences of the accident;
- long-term epidemiological studies, based on reliable exposure and clinical records, to identify the types of tumours in the exposed population and developmental disorders among those irradiated prenatally, and to determine the rate of induction by radiation dose;
- foundations laid for possible studies of genetic effects in future generations.

To achieve these aims, IPHECA identified a number of tasks that were necessary to give assistance to health care services and to facilitate the collection of medical data that could be useful for research. These tasks were:
- provision of essential medical equipment and supplies, and training of medical and ancillary staff;
- continued refinement, through retrospective studies, of the assessment of the nature and extent of radioactive contamination from the accident, including individual doses;
- careful selection of control groups;
- establishment and continued updating of registers of exposed persons and controls, with links to databases of vital statistics, medical records and other information;
- continued supply of equipment, reagents and spares for the programme until the countries concerned were in a position to provide these;
- effective and sustained exchange of information and experience among research centres by means of meetings and visits.

It was neither necessary nor feasible to start all these activities simultaneously. IPHECA was implemented in phases according to the health consequences identified, the capacity of the national and local authorities and the resources available. The initial work consisted of five pilot projects, each addressing a high-priority health need. The pilot projects related to the following:
- selected thyroid diseases, including thyroid cancer, among children (the thyroid project);
- leukaemia and related blood diseases (the haematology project);
- brain damage from prenatal exposure (the brain damage *in utero* project);

19

- management of epidemiological registries (the epidemiological registry project);
- oral health in Belarus.

Each project included specific activities (development of standardized protocols for the three countries, procurement of equipment and supplies, professional training both on-site and abroad) and was underpinned by common support measures (physical and biological dosimetry, communications, dissemination of information, general diagnostic services, management support).

In each rayon, teams of specialists screened the population for selected health disorders. Thorough medical examinations were carried out at the oblast and national levels. The IPHECA projects, which were of limited duration, have paved the way for long-term activity by establishing standardized procedures and scientific methods, and by providing the necessary equipment and training.

Dosimetry

Determination of the degree and extent of radioactive contamination and assessment of individual and population doses were essential for the IPHECA pilot projects. This involved the reconstruction, recording and verification of thyroid doses, and estimation of the contributions of internal and external exposure to both the individual effective dose and the collective dose.

To support existing dosimetric methods and the development of new techniques, specialists from the three countries were trained at institutions in Germany, Japan and the United Kingdom. This training resulted in use of the latest techniques for physical and biological dosimetry.

Central dose registries have been established in each of the three countries to record dose contributions from all relevant exposure sources for individuals. Demographic details, contamination levels and types of dosimetric technique are also included in the registries. Each central registry has a number of local databases containing information on the types of radionuclides and activity levels in the contaminated areas and individual doses determined by direct measurements. Dose measurement techniques include thermoluminescent dosimetry for external irradiation and whole-body counting and radioiodine measurement for incorporated radioisotopes, mainly caesium and iodine. The results are used for retrospective dose determination and prediction of future exposures using statistical models.

Thyroid project

The IPHECA thyroid project began in 1992. One of its main purposes was to strengthen local capabilities for the early detection of thyroid disorders, and it was therefore integrated into national programmes dealing with the health effects of the Chernobyl accident.

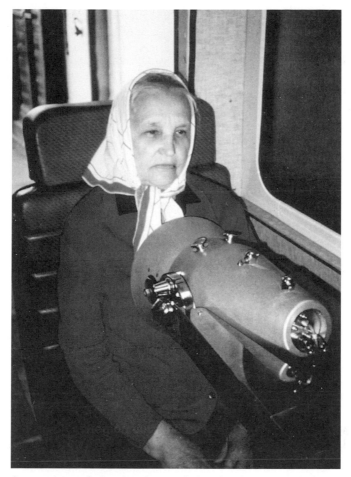

A member of the local population having a whole-body radiation count (photo WHO/IAEA/P. Pavlicek).

Because serious thyroid diseases were suspected, screening programmes were implemented with a standardized protocol to detect and characterize thyroid cancers, benign tumours, autoimmune thyroiditis and hypothyroidism. These disorders can be caused by radiation and their incidence might therefore increase with time, especially among children living in areas of high radioactive contamination. The protocol was finalized by experts from the three countries in collaboration with WHO and other international specialists. It took account of local financial constraints and the need to collect the data within a limited time. More than 50 000 children born after 1971 and before 1987, who lived in contaminated areas, were screened according to the project protocol and the results were compared with those for children living in uncontaminated areas.

WHO provided 20 ultrasound units for use in hospitals and in the field, as well as instruments and kits for radio-immunoassays and enzyme-immunoassays to determine thyroid function and to monitor the progress of cancer treatment.

Staff were trained, both locally by equipment suppliers and abroad by specialist institutes in France, Germany, Japan and the United Kingdom, in the use of the new equipment and in ultrasonography techniques, hormone analysis and reconstruction of thyroid doses.

Findings

To be able to link any health consequences to radiation exposure it is necessary to know the doses received by patients. Thyroid doses are measured in grays (Gy), which are the units of absorbed dose or of energy imparted by ionizing radiation to a unit mass of tissue. One gray corresponds to one joule per kilogram. When exposure is to a mixture of radiations (e.g. alpha and gamma rays with different effects), their contribution is weighted to obtain the equivalent dose measured in sieverts (Sv). A further weighting is made when the irradiation is non-uniform to account for different susceptibilities of tissues and organs (e.g. thyroid versus lung). The result is the effective dose, also measured in sieverts.

While the dose data given below come from direct measurements on people, the information in most cases is still incomplete. The highest thyroid doses were recorded in the Gomel and Mogilev oblasts of Belarus, at distances up to 300 km from Chernobyl. These oblasts had caesium-137 contamination higher than 555 kBq/m^2. Children aged up to two years had the highest exposure. The recorded thyroid doses were up to 50 Gy, with about 1% of children evacuated from the heavily contaminated areas having doses exceeding 10 Gy. Of the children who contracted thyroid cancer, 66% had radiation doses of less than 0.3 Gy, 22% had 0.3–1 Gy, and 12% had 1 Gy or more. Adult thyroid radiation doses were calculated to be in the range 0.1–50 Gy.

The highest thyroid doses recorded in the Russian Federation were measured in children aged 1–3 years in Bryansk and Kaluga oblasts. In some cases these were 10 Gy or higher with the average absorbed doses ranging between 10 mGy and 2.2 Gy in children of different age groups. Adult doses were as high as 1–2 Gy.

In Ukraine, the highest thyroid doses were detected in people living in Chernigov, Kiev and Zhitomir oblasts near the Chernobyl reactor site. Direct measurements of iodine-131 activity in the thyroid showed that children received average doses of 1–2 Gy, with individual doses reaching up to 30 Gy in the most contaminated rayons. Adult doses were 2–8 times lower.

An increase in the incidence of childhood thyroid cancer has been one of the major health consequences of the Chernobyl accident. Before the accident the annual incidence of childhood thyroid cancer in Belarus was about one per million. By 1994 it had risen to 36 per million children. More than half of these childhood cancers have occurred in the Gomel oblast which is immediately to the north of the Chernobyl site and under the path of the initial fallout cloud. Annual incidence rates in Gomel reached more than 100 per million children in 1994, a hundredfold increase over the rates before the accident. Table 3 summarizes the extent and incidence of childhood thyroid cancer in the three countries.

Table 3

Childhood thyroid cancer 1986–1994 in Belarus, the Russian Federation (Bryansk and Kaluga oblasts) and Ukraine

| | Number of cases per year | | | | | | | | | |
	1986	1987	1988	1989	1990	1991	1992	1993	1994	Total
Belarus	2	4	5	7	29	59	66	79	82	333
Russian Federation	0	1	0	0	2	0	4	6	11	24
Ukraine	8	7	8	11	26	22	47	42	37*	208*

| | Incidence (rounded) per million children | | | | | | | | |
	1986	1987	1988	1989	1990	1991	1992	1993	1994
Belarus	0.9	1.7	2.2	3.0	13	26	28	34	36
Russian Federation	0.0	2.0	0.0	0.0	4.0	0.0	8.0	12	22
Ukraine	0.7	0.6	0.7	0.9	2.2	1.8	3.9	3.5	3.1*

Note: * = incomplete number
Belarus has 2.3 million children, Ukraine has 12 million and the Bryansk and Kaluga oblasts of the Russian Federation have 500 000.

The annual incidence of thyroid cancer in children in Ukraine from 1981 to 1985 was 0.4–0.5 per million. The incidence of childhood thyroid cancers significantly increased to 2.2 cases per million in 1990, 1.8 cases in 1991, 3.9 in 1992, 3.5 in 1993, and at least 3.1 in 1994. This represents an approximate eightfold increase over levels registered before the accident. This increase occurred mainly in northern Ukraine where the highest radioiodine contaminations were found and more than 60% of all childhood thyroid cancer cases were registered.

Thyroid cancer in children in 1992–1994 ranged between 20.0 and 24.5 cases per million children in the Kiev oblast. The incidence in the Chernigov oblast was between 15.4 and 35.1, in the Zhitomir oblast it was 10.0–16.0, in Cherkassy it was 6.7–13.1 and in Rovno it was 7.0–17.0. In the city of Kiev, this indicator reached 10.0–18.0 cases per million children. Before the Chernobyl accident, childhood thyroid cancer was very low in these oblasts (except for Cherkassy). Eight out of 10 of the children treated for cancer in these regions had radioiodine doses to the thyroid of no more than 1 Gy. However, 20% of the children had doses of 1–1.5 Gy.

In the Russian Federation, the increase in childhood thyroid cancers occurred later, was at a lower incidence than in Belarus and Ukraine, and was confined to Bryansk and Kaluga. The annual incidence of thyroid cancer in children in these oblasts before the accident was about 0.5 per million. In 1994, the incidence had increased to 22 cases per million children. A positive correlation was detected between the thyroid exposure dose and the incidence of thyroid cancer in children and adolescents living in areas with different levels of caesium-137 contamination.

More than 95% of the thyroid cancers reported in children in the affected areas of all three countries were highly invasive, spreading both within the thyroid gland and into surrounding soft tissues, lymph nodes, blood vessels and the lungs. Normally thyroid cancer can be successfully removed with good prospects of complete recovery. However, because these cancers were highly invasive, a few of the children died. Most cases of childhood thyroid cancers in Belarus and more than 60% in Ukraine were verified by international experts. The diagnoses were confirmed in virtually all cases.

Screening, especially with the use of ultrasound, may have increased the detection of cancers, particularly small and occult tumours. In Ukraine up to half the cases of childhood thyroid cancer were revealed using ultrasound screening, though in the three countries combined only 12% of childhood cancers were detected by this method alone. Although there were reported increases in thyroid cancer in adolescents and adults, in these groups screening for thyroid cancer and awareness that it might occur may have led to cases being revealed that would otherwise have remained undiagnosed, and therefore the reported increases may not be wholly due to radiation.

The increase in thyroid pathology which started some four years after the accident, and its predominance in regions affected by the fallout, strongly suggest that exposure to radioactive iodine was the primary cause. However, this has not been unequivocally proved since, for short-lived isotopes such as those of iodine, it is difficult to estimate radiation doses to the thyroid well after the exposure has taken place. Inhalation in the early stages of the release of radioactivity may have contributed significantly to the dose to the thyroid, particularly in the areas near Chernobyl.

Diseases such as autoimmune thyroiditis, nodular goitre and hypothyroidism show no reliable signs of increase, although they have been less intensely studied.

Apart from endemic goitre, in areas where dietary iodine is deficient, as in most of the areas affected by the Chernobyl accident, there tends to be a greater prevalence of the follicular forms of thyroid cancer. There is no evidence to suggest, however, that iodine deficiency alone could have caused the increase in thyroid cancer in children.

The data suggest that the large increases in thyroid cancer in children are related to radiation exposure, though further epidemiological study is required.

Haematology project

This project was established to detect and treat leukaemia and related blood disorders in the population of around 270 000 in the Strictly Controlled Zones of the three countries. Rigorous epidemiological methods were used for the detection of what was expected to be a very small increase.

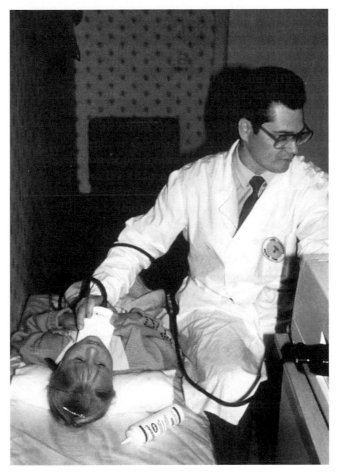

A child being tested for thyroid radioactivity (photo WHO/ IAEA/V. Mouchkin).

Health care institutions at both local (rayon) and oblast levels cooperated in the detection and treatment of blood disorders, using a protocol devised for this purpose. Equipment such as blood cell analysers, flow cytometers, blood bio-chemistry analysers and microscopes was acquired so that advanced haema-tological investigations could be carried out. Since reconstruction of doses by physical and biological methods was indispensable for all patients with a blood disorder thought to be caused by radiation exposure, equipment was provided for physical dosimetry (thermoluminescent dosimeters, gamma spectrometers) and biological dosimetry (machines for cytogenetic analysis, electron spin reso-nance spectrometers for tooth enamel analysis). Specialists from the three countries were trained both locally and abroad.

Findings

To evaluate the association of radiation exposure with leukaemia and other haematological diseases, it is necessary to determine the radiation doses received by the whole body, the bone marrow and the fetus. Exposure is almost entirely due to caesium-137 which is received through fresh vegetables and milk. Radiation from radioisotopes of strontium and plutonium amounts to no more than 5% of the total dose. Since the pattern of fallout was irregular, measurements of caesium activity had to be made at a large number of places.

The average accumulated dose to residents of most contaminated settlements in Belarus, as of late 1993, was estimated to be not more than 5 mSv per year. Lower average annual doses have been found in the most contaminated settlements of the Russian Federation and Ukraine. Since these are average doses, significantly higher individual doses from both internal and external exposure have been recorded.

In the course of the haematology project, a number of blood disorders were revealed and verified in areas with caesium-137 contamination levels of 555 kBq/m²:

- In Belarus from 1979 to 1985, there were 681 cases (97 per year) but in the post-accident period 1986–1993 there was a total of 824 cases (103 per year).
- In the Bryansk oblast of the Russian Federation from 1979 to 1985, there were 208 cases (30 per year), while during 1986–1993 there was a total of 288 cases (36 per year).
- In Ukraine from 1980 to 1985, there were 146 cases (24 per year) but during 1986–1993 there was a total of 254 cases (32 per year).

While this shows an upward trend in the three countries after the accident, the general morbidity for leukaemia and other blood disorders did not significantly differ in this period. This was because there was a slow upward trend in morbidity in both the contaminated and the uncontaminated areas. Comparison of morbidity in the areas with different levels of radioactive contamination produced no significant differences.

The incidence of childhood leukaemia did not change significantly after the accident compared with the period before 1986 and there were no deviations in age distribution or correlations of disease types with dose.

Thus the results obtained so far show no changes in morbidity which could be linked to the effects of radiation. However, plans have been made to continue detection and registration of cases and to use case–control studies to identify possible links between individual exposure dose and risk of disease.

An important outcome of the IPHECA project is the significant improvement of diagnostic facilities in health services and of qualifications of medical personnel. This may have led to more effective early detection and diagnosis of leukaemia and other blood disorders.

Brain damage *in utero* project

This project set out to examine all children born within a year of the accident to women evacuated from within 30 km of the reactor site or to women living in the Strictly Controlled Zones. Children born in uncontaminated areas were matched for age, socioeconomic background, residential environment and educational level, and served as controls for the project. A protocol was adopted for the investigations which included assessments of mental retardation and cognitive impairment, anthropometric measurements, neurological and endocrinological assessments, and brain-mapping. The project included provision for training both locally and abroad, and for the supply of scientific equipment such as apparatus for the computerized analysis of electroencephalograms.

In all, 4210 children were examined in the three countries, as follows:

- in Belarus, 906 children in the contaminated areas (exposed group) and 962 in the "clean" rayons (control group);
- in the Russian Federation, 725 children in the contaminated areas and 300 in the clean rayons;
- in Ukraine, 558 children in the contaminated areas (including 115 children and their mothers evacuated from Pripyat and Chernobyl) and 759 in the clean rayons.

Findings

The preliminary results of the investigations in the three countries suggest the following:

- the incidence of mental retardation in the exposed children was higher than in the control group;
- there was an upward trend in behavioural disorders and emotional problems in exposed children;
- the incidence of borderline nervous and psychological disorders in the parents of the exposed group was higher than that in the controls.

On the basis of investigations conducted so far, it is impossible to reach any definitive conclusions about the relationship between a rise in the number of mentally retarded children and the ionizing radiation due to the Chernobyl accident. The results obtained are difficult to interpret and require verification. The stress and concern of parents, for instance, could have influenced the results. While the infrastructure for research has been established, it is necessary to continue well planned epidemiological investigations and dosimetric follow-up.

Epidemiological registry project

Vital statistics and health and socioeconomic records must be complete, consistent, reliable and accessible if a population's state of health is to be assessed. Details of radiation exposure are also needed.

The Chernobyl epidemiological registries were established in Belarus, the Russian Federation and Ukraine. Registration and medical follow-up was mandatory for four main groups:

Group 1 — accident recovery workers

Group 2 — population evacuated from the areas with most contamination (>1480 kBq/m²)

Group 3 — residents of contaminated areas (>555 kBq/m²)

Group 4 — children of persons in groups 1–3.

Data collected in the rayons and oblasts are kept in local registries and also sent to the national registry. Data in the national Chernobyl registries include the following:

- passport information and primary registration group;
- place of residence, activities at the time of the accident, type of work (taken from the registration card);
- radiation dose, if known;
- medical information, periodically updated, covering all diagnosed diseases and types of treatment at rayon, oblast and national levels.

The epidemiological registry project was started in 1991 to assist existing national registration programmes systematically with provision of computers, development of software for data processing, training of personnel and quality control of data. The project was integrated into national programmes and the Chernobyl registries became components of the national registries in Belarus, the Russian Federation and Ukraine.

A single general record chart was developed on the basis of the thyroid, haematology and epidemiological registry pilot projects to gather data for effective in-depth monitoring of the health status of the population.

The registries include data on indicators of morbidity, disease incidence and life expectancy, and allow a comparative analysis to be made of radiation and non-radiation risk factors. A special software package was devised to allow standard analyses of data.

Oral health project

Deterioration of oral health, and particularly dryness of the mouth, were common complaints received by the medical teams in the contaminated areas, especially in Belarus. While the problem was unlikely to be related to radiation exposure at the dose levels received, the complaints were frequent and, because of anxiety about possible radiation exposure, a specific project on oral health was developed in Belarus. The objective of this project was to determine whether there was a relationship between radiation exposure and oral and dental disorders. Some 5000 subjects in the Strictly Controlled Zones were enlisted in the project and samples of tooth enamel were used for individual dose assessment.

Findings

The incidence of diseases of the oral mucosa and periodontal and dental tissues was almost identical among residents of the contaminated (>555 kBq/m²) and clean rayons of Belarus. In some age groups (15, 18 and 34–44 years), more frequent complaints of dryness in the mouth were noted in the residents of the Strictly Controlled Zones. Inadequate oral hygiene may, however, be a more substantial factor than radiation.

The 12-month prevention programmes, under which young people aged 15–19 in the contaminated areas of Mogilev oblast used toothbrushes and fluoridated toothpaste, proved to be highly effective in preventing the development of caries and reducing dental plaque to the normal level.

7

Future work

IPHECA has contributed significantly to the improvement of diagnostic and therapeutic capabilities in Belarus, the Russian Federation and Ukraine. International support is still required for medical equipment and supplies, the maintenance of imported equipment, and information exchange with the world scientific community. The maintenance and updating of the epidemiological registries will grow in importance as the long-term effects of the accident emerge. The registries will require increasing attention as the people exposed to the Chernobyl fallout grow older. Some may migrate, making them more difficult to trace.

The health studies have made an essential contribution to assessment of the impact of the accident and to development of realistic plans for emergency preparedness and response in the case of similar accidents in the future. The studies have also added to our knowledge of the risks from activities that involve exposure to radiation, thus making it possible, among other things, to compare better the risks of different forms of energy production. These are long-term research activities that will require a great deal of effort along with continuing resources, both locally and internationally. It is imperative to take advantage of this unique opportunity to increase our knowledge of the long-term effects of low-level radiation exposure.

In March 1994, IPHECA's management committee considered the future activities of the programme. The committee endorsed a proposal by the representatives of the three countries that IPHECA support three major initiatives relating to accident recovery workers, dose reconstruction and thyroid diseases. It further recommended that some IPHECA funds be reallocated as seed money for these activities. In addition, the committee recommended that guidelines be prepared on public health action following nuclear accidents, based on the experience of the follow-up to the Chernobyl accident and the implementation of IPHECA. Each of these proposed activities is briefly described below.

Accident recovery workers

The Russian Federation, with the support of Belarus and Ukraine, has proposed that accident recovery workers should be the subject of a specific IPHECA project. The project would aim to investigate and mitigate the health effects of the accident on these persons. There are some 800 000 of these accident recovery workers, including about 350 000 in the Russian Federation alone. They received various doses of radiation, with about one-third of them estimated to have received doses in excess of 200 mGy. Early reports indicate increased morbidity and mortality among them. Numerous investigations have been carried out and efforts to alleviate their health problems and to rehabilitate them have been made by national and local authorities. These are still continuing, but a more systematic approach with more technical support is necessary.

An international consultation on the Chernobyl accident recovery workers was convened in St Petersburg in 1994 by the Russian Ministry of Health and Medical Industry and WHO. The consultation reviewed the status of programmes dealing with accident recovery workers and discussed ways to improve and strengthen these efforts. Participants agreed that the primary purpose of the IPHECA project should be to assist the health care systems, focusing on the strengthening and coordination of efforts in the three countries to provide diagnosis, treatment and rehabilitation of the accident recovery workers and their families. The second but very important purpose would be to lay the foundation for research into health effects by enabling systematic acquisition and management of data from national health care programmes and other sources. It is likely that the project will be extended to other nations of the former USSR with sizeable populations of accident recovery workers and also to nations which have large numbers of immigrants from the affected areas.

Dose reconstruction

The accurate retrospective calculation of individual radiation doses is vital for estimating the risk of radiation-induced disorders and for conducting relevant epidemiological and other research. While there have been substantial dose reconstruction efforts, including some as part of the IPHECA pilot projects, common protocols are not being used and much more work needs to be completed. At present there are only a few laboratories worldwide that specialize in techniques for determining individual radiation doses. An IPHECA project on dose reconstruction would facilitate international cooperation so that available technologies for dose reconstruction could be compared and the best method or methods could be developed. The management committee emphasized that the project should be well coordinated with current bilateral dose reconstruction activities such as those sponsored by the European Union, the United States and other countries.

The broad terms of reference for the dose reconstruction project would be as follows:
1. To develop a common methodology for reconstruction of doses received by persons exposed to radiation in contaminated areas.
2. To reconstruct internal and external radiation doses.
3. To compile an inventory of verified doses for people in Belarus, the Russian Federation and Ukraine.
4. To strengthen dose monitoring programmes in the three countries.
5. To provide data to research programmes.

Thyroid disease

Further efforts to study the incidence of thyroid diseases and to treat patients are clearly necessary. Consequently the management committee endorsed the proposal that the pilot project on the thyroid be extended and expanded to include reconstruction of thyroid dose, continuation of surveillance of populations covered by the pilot project, expansion of surveillance to other areas, investigation of the etiology of thyroid cancer in children, study of thyroid cancer in adults, and the local manufacture of diagnostic kits. As an initial effort in this direction, the management committee supported an initiative by the WHO Regional Office for Europe (the International Thyroid Project) which, in cooperation with the International Agency for Research on Cancer, will address the thyroid cancer problem in Belarus. The aims of this project are to identify groups most at risk, to promote a better understanding of the nature and cause of thyroid cancer, and to assist Belarus in managing the disease.

The International Thyroid Project has already received funding from Switzerland. It will be implemented through a WHO Collaborating Centre to be designated in Minsk, Belarus, and through seven international collaborating centres in France, Germany, Italy, Japan, Sweden, Switzerland and the United Kingdom. A project office has been opened in Minsk and a project officer appointed. Some initial funding for the project has been reallocated from IPHECA funds and the WHO Regional Office for Europe is seeking further funding as a matter of urgency.

Guidelines on public health action

Much new information has been obtained about the actions that should or should not be taken to safeguard people's health and to investigate and treat the effects on health following a nuclear accident. Guidelines will be prepared which will include cost–benefit analyses and will deal with issues such as whether screening the population is cost–effective, what emergency measures should be taken, and what approaches are best for investigating the health consequences in populations. Other international organizations concerned with the consequences of nuclear accidents have expressed interest in cooperating in this work.

8

Conclusions

While the main objective of IPHECA has been to support programmes concerned with radiation-related health effects, the national programmes have investigated all possible health consequences of the accident. These have included health effects considered to be related to the stress that resulted from being evacuated from home and fear of possible future radiation-induced health damage. The main conclusions that can be drawn from the national programmes, including the IPHECA pilot projects, are the following:

- Psychosocial effects, believed to be unrelated to direct radiation exposure, resulted from the lack of information immediately after the accident, the stress and trauma of compulsory relocation to less contaminated areas, the break in social ties among community members, and the fear that radiation exposure could cause health damage in the future. National registries recorded significant increases in many diseases that are not related to radiation. This is an important health consequence of the Chernobyl accident in view of the size of the population affected and the burden on the health care systems.

- The Chernobyl accident resulted in a sharp increase in thyroid cancer, especially among children living in the contaminated areas. The total number of thyroid cancer cases reported among children (aged 0–14 at the time of diagnosis) in the three countries in the post-accident period was, by the end of 1994, 565 (333 in Belarus, 24 in the Russian Federation, 208 in Ukraine). An increase in childhood thyroid cancer to about 100 times the pre-accident levels was recorded in the Gomel oblast of Belarus which lay in the direct path of the initial cloud of radioactive fallout.

- There was no significant increase in the incidence of leukaemia or other blood disorders. This may be expected given the short time frame of this study. However, since the peak in the incidence of blood disorders may occur more than 10 years after the accident, long-term studies of these diseases are needed.

- Some evidence was found to suggest retarded mental development and deviations in behavioural and emotional reactions in a small group of children exposed to radiation *in utero*. The extent to which radiation may have contributed to such psychological changes cannot be determined because of the absence of individual dosimetry data.

- The types and distribution of oral diseases observed in the residents of contaminated areas of Belarus were the same as those of the residents of uncontaminated areas.

WHO purchased and supplied to the three countries equipment and medical supplies to the value of about US$16 000 000. The balance of the funding for the pilot projects was expended in programme support, scientific meetings, training courses in foreign research and clinical institutions for 200 specialists, and seed money for continuing IPHECA activities. Specialists from the three countries were involved with international experts in developing investigation programmes and establishing unified projects.

IPHECA has rendered substantial assistance to the national health care systems of Belarus, the Russian Federation and Ukraine in alleviating the health consequences of the Chernobyl accident. The results obtained in the course of the IPHECA pilot projects have considerably improved scientific knowledge of the effects of a radiation accident on human health. This knowledge will serve as the basis for guidelines for planning and developing further investigations.

The chronology of the Chernobyl accident

26 April 1986	Reactor accident occurred at 01:23. Government commission formed.
27 April 1986	Town of Pripyat evacuated.
3 & 6 May 1986	"Temporary permissible levels" introduced for drinking-water and food consumption.
May 1986	"Temporary dose limits" for the population set at 100 mSv annual total dose (combined internal and external) during the first year after the accident.
30 May 1986	Revision of "temporary permissible levels" for drinking-water and food.
July 1986	First contamination map completed.
November 1986	Completion of sarcophagus around disabled reactor.
1987	"Temporary dose limits" for the population reduced to 30 mSv annual total dose for the second year after the accident.
April 1987	Completion of work begun in May 1986 to protect the water system.
December 1987	Revision of the "temporary permissible levels" for drinking-water and food established 30 May 1986.
1988	"Temporary dose limits" for the population reduced to 25 mSv annual total dose for 1988 and 1989.
October 1988	The 350 mSv lifetime dose recommended by NCRP.
March 1989	Radioactive contamination maps officially published in the three republics.
October 1989	IAEA assistance requested by Soviet Government.
Early 1990	WHO requested by Soviet Ministry of Health to develop an international programme of assistance.

May 1991   International Chernobyl Project completed through IAEA.

May 1991   IPHECA established at WHO by agreement with the Soviet Government.

April 1992   Ministers of health of Belarus, the Russian Federation and Ukraine and the Director-General of WHO agree to collaborate on IPHECA.